Green Pigs in Autumn

By Anna Mould

Copyright © 2024 by Anna Mould

All rights reserved. No part of this book may be reproduced or used in any manner without written permission on the copyright owner except for use in quotations in a book review.

First paperback edition 2024

Cover design by Katie Brookes Illustrations

ISBN 9798333645104

www.annamouldauthor.co.uk

To my peri-sisters across the globe. Keep your fire burning bright!

<u>Introduction - am I alone in this?</u>

One of my reasons for writing this book was to share my experience of midlife and perimenopause, so that other women would know that they are not alone. I have felt very alone at times, isolated by my feelings and paranoia. Until I connected with Sophie Cartledge at Hormones On The Blink, I honestly thought I was going mad, losing my mind, that my life was about to implode. If I hadn't known about her and the work she does, I wonder how the last year would have panned out. Would I still be in the grips of anxiety and rage? Would my relationships have survived? Would I still be employed?

As I wrote, I realised that I hadn't heard the voices of other women and their experiences, and I wanted to reach out in a bid to see "what's it like for others?" I wanted to know how other women felt about this time of life, whether they had any expectations of this new chapter, how were they handling it? I put a shout out via social media with a simple Google form to collect their responses. I am so grateful to the women who took the time to tell me their thoughts and feelings about this tumultuous time - I feel truly honoured that they shared their experiences with me in the spirit of simply spreading awareness and sharing with others so that they may be better equipped going forward.

What follows is an overview of what they told me.

Respondents were between the ages of 39 and 60 (average age 48) and had been experiencing symptoms of perimenopause for between one and ten years (average four and a half years). 42% of respondents were still experiencing regular periods. When asked whether they had known what to expect in the years leading up to menopause, 89% responded "no." I asked what symptoms they had been expecting, and responses varied:

"I didn't know what to expect. Hot flushes, as that's what everyone talks about and I haven't even had them."

"Hot flushes and periods changing/stopping."

"Hot flushes and night sweats."

"Memory loss, weight gain, hot sweats."

Moodiness, memory changes, brain fog, being tearful, anger, palpitations, dizziness, bladder problems.

"Being a bit of an arse."

"Going a bit weird and mental."

"Sense of debilitating 'what is the point?'"

I asked what symptoms have been unexpected:

"My sex drive is rising, not dropping."

"Mood swings were an eye opener!"

"My mood swings and emotions seem heightened: sometimes my anger/irritation feels almost irrational, or I become very weepy quite easily (often over things like tv commercials or even dog videos), and recently I could FEEL anxiety coursing through me in this oppressive wave (I don't normally suffer too much with anxiety, or at least not to this level, but this particular day I felt buried under it, just this overwhelming sense of restlessness, despair, worry, inadequacy, a feeling of being trapped and hopeless. Luckily, it passed after a day or two, but it was very much tied to hormonal fluctuations. It sort of scares me thinking that as my body continues to change that these episodes may be longer lasting.)"

"The weight has gone on everywhere, but esp my belly and thighs, and now my clothes don't fit and I feel terrible (and my workouts are harder because I weigh more... it's a vicious cycle.) And I just feel like the weight will not come off, even if I'm doing "the right things" and living a healthy lifestyle."

Mood swings and brain fog, anxiety, palpitations, low mood, achy body and extreme tiredness, bloating, very heavy and irregular periods (sometimes lasting months), lack of libido, lack of motivation, lack of confidence, loss of interest in hobbies, loss of enthusiasm for life in general. Urinary incontinence, extreme pain in feet, itchy skin.

"Age of onset. Menopause or any aspect of women's health were never discussed or mentioned by my mother. 2 old brothers and all male cousins. "Taboo" subject, even talking about periods."

When I asked which three symptoms had had the biggest impact on their daily lives, each of the symptoms was mentioned by at least one respondent. The hardest comment to read was this one:

"Wanting to escape my life so badly, the feeling there is no point in going on."

Every person born with a uterus is going to go through this transition, and the impact on the individuals needs to be recognised, acknowledged and treated seriously. It is not "just" hormones changing. It's not just physical changes. It affects our mental health and well-being, to the point where some individuals see no way forward. I hope with all hope that the person writing this last comment has the support that they need (all responses were anonymous).

I asked whether they were using hormone replacement therapy (HRT), and only 42% said that they were. I enquired into the reasons individuals were not using HRT, and some of the responses were surprising, some made me sad, others made me angry:

"Despite having a blood test at 38 showing low testosterone levels, I was told I was too young for HRT and to come back when I was fifty."

"I guess I'm not sure my symptoms have gotten "bad enough" yet? I've been reading up on it, though, and have even been more alert to the idea of adaptogen supplements (most of which, however, I worry are actually just scams because women's health --especially women's reproductive and hormonal health-- has been ignored, devalued, & ignored/not studied the way it OBVIOUSLY should have been (which PISSES ME TF OFF!!!!) and so now there's this whole untapped market that scammers are trying to make a quick buck off of because a whole ignored gender is now desperate to be heard, understood, and helped, and they're taking advantage rather than actually helping to solve a problem. See? Told you it pisses me off. haha)"

Nervous about the risks and how their body would react. Lack of information and access.

"Had a blood test and was told I wasn't menopausal."

"Too embarrassed to go to the doctor."

"Caused more problems"

I asked respondents what they had tried or were implementing to help with symptoms other than HRT.

Exercise (walking, gym, yoga, swimming), limiting dairy intake, taking supplements ("Womanopause", multivitamins, D3, marine collagen, magnesium, cod liver oil, B complex, iron, glucosamine sulphate), regular sleep schedule, meditation, hypnosis, eating well, "Advil for aches and pains", "Fem Magnet", talking, "taking time for myself."

Which did they find most effective? Exercise seemed to come out on top, as well as taking time out and talking with other women. Most comments said that nothing really had a huge impact, but HRT "really helped" some respondents.

I asked them what they wished they had been told before perimenopause began:

"That it's OK, it's all normal and there is actually so much help and information out then once you look for it or talk to the right people."

"That it even existed and what all the symptoms are."

"I don't know. I guess I really just wish it had been more studied so it wasn't such an unknown entity for womankind."

"Oestrogen is safe and effective."

"How difficult it would make generally coping."

"That what I am going through is OK."

"Everything. In a leaflet. Even might get symptoms."

"How many symptoms can impact daily life, anxiety."

"Everything and it's ok to talk …"

"Nothing, I am more than able to research this myself if needed."

"About how heavy bleeding can be."

"I had no idea it would affect me mentally. I have had to leave a job because I wasn't doing well mentally and physically. I burnt out and assumed it was the stressful work but I can see now it was a combination of the mental and physical effects of the perimenopause."

"The truth about what to expect and who to speak to."

"The truth about how varied the symptoms could be and that I wasn't having a midlife crisis!"

"How overwhelming it is and how much you don't feel like yourself."

"That I could and should have asked for hrt much much sooner and spoken to my GP / Health professional. Assumed it was all anxiety related."

"What actually happens."

"All of it.....nobody used to talk about it. Glad things are changing now. A senior manager at my work (a man) took part in a podcast about menopause which I thought was brilliant."

"I think any woman approaching 40 should be made aware of the change beginning soon."

Finally, I asked how they felt about this time of their life, and the responses resonated strongly with me...

"I'm not sure how I feel about it really as it was all brought on due to surgery not out of natural causes."

"Very negative, I feel ruled by my hormones and personally can't wait to get through the other side of the menopause."

"That's an interesting question. I guess I have mixed feelings. It's a little scary in some ways because it feels to a degree like a long period of being out of control? Like I'll be at the mercy of whatever my hormones dictate at any given time. That feels scary and unpleasant. Just the small tastes of it I've had so far leave me not wanting more of that. On the other hand, the idea of not having periods at some point feels freeing. (Though the thought of lower libido, vaginal dryness, possible more frequent urinary infections sounds like a fucking nightmare, to the point where maybe the devil I know--bleeding--is less terrible after all?) I don't know. It kind of makes me feel old, too, which I also have mixed feelings about. I definitely don't want to have more children, but I don't want to start worrying about things like bone loss. On the other hand, I do like the sense of community I feel with other women navigating the same things. I feel like we're more open about discussing our cycles, our symptoms, our womanhood than in some earlier stages of life. (Or maybe that's not accurate. Maybe it's the same amount but different topics? IDK. But it FEELS more like a club.) If I had to choose, though, I guess I'd mostly say negative?"

"Positive...happy to be over the worst and onto the next stage of my life."

"It's exhausting and I want it over."

"I'm not a happy person, wish I didn't have to go through this."

"I feel there is more to come."

"Mostly negative."

"Negative as getting older is embarrassing, people judge you and dismiss you so easily."

"Positive, I am very happy in both my personal and professional life."

"Negative at the moment. Impacts quality of life."

"Presently I loathe it! I feel old, fat, washed up, lacking in energy and unattractive. I'm constantly scared of everything and feel as though I get through every day at work by the skin of my teeth."

"Negative. Lack of understanding and lack of support from professionals."

"I just feel useless now & stupid as I doubt everything I do. I'm still alive so that is the only positive I see about myself at the moment but it's not a quality or true life."

"Mixed feelings as I don't always know how I am going to be."

"With hrt it's all good."

"Negative .. no longer feel like myself anymore."

"Neither really, it just is what it is. I am generally happy."

"NEGATIVE......"

I left space for any other comments:

"Best wishes with your book! Hope my experiences are helpful to you in some way."

"If menopause was suffered by men, hormones would be available over the counter. Trying to get access to doctors to discuss treatment is nearly impossible and time consuming; at a point in life where women don't have the time to devote to their own health. Recently watched the Davina Mcall documentary, really informative."

"We need more menopause specialists in all doctors' surgeries. I know I'm not on the right dose /HRT, but it's too much hassle to sort out. If I could afford to go private I would."

"People are very unkind, it's a difficult time to go through, your emotions are brutal."

"I'm due to have an endometrial ablation to sort the problem."

"I'm sad that I feel so negative about everything currently. It stops me from enjoying work and hobbies."

"I had a blood test 2 years ago and got told I am peri but have had no follow up or support given to me. I also have osteoporosis which has been linked to this but have had no follow up for this either."

"I can't wait to find the right combo of HRT to make me feel human again!"

"Thanks for raising awareness, it can only be a good thing."

Reading the responses was bittersweet - I am definitely not alone, but so many women are struggling and suffering. The lack of awareness of perimemopause and menopause impacts not only on the individual, but also their loved ones, their colleagues, employers and society more widely. We feel like we are failing in some way, no good anymore, unable to function at work or at home. And the societal view of older women is that they are "past their prime."

As a woman nearing fifty years of age (and mentally still not feeling like an adult yet!) I don't want the next few years of my life to be dominated by doom and gloom, of becoming decrepit, losing my usefulness in the world. I feel like I am coming back to me, rediscovering myself, and at a point when the years of experience and wisdom can come into their own. My fire has not gone out yet, there are plenty of sparks left, plenty of things to be excited and passionate about, plans to be made.

I just need to figure out what and how.

I am not past my prime. Older women are coming into their strength and power, when we can finally think about ourselves first. But, seriously, what the fuck is perimenopause??!!

<u>9th October 2022</u>

Dear reader,

It has been so long since I last sat to write to you. I think my last letter was in January. 2022 has been a strange, tumultuous time. War in Ukraine still goes on. A change in government leadership has sent the country into chaos, and has set millions on the path of poverty. Queen Elizabeth II passed away aged 96, leading to a nation in mourning,

Overseas, the US has revoked legislation which ensured women had access to safe abortions.

In Iran, on the day our Queen died, a young woman was killed for not wearing her veil.

Flooding in Pakistan. Storms and other natural disasters across the globe remind us how fragile our home is.

For me, my word for 2022 was "trust" - and, boy, was that challenged! We started the year knowing we had to move home (not through choice, and completely unexpected). I had to trust that we would find a new home, which we did and it is so lovely (although I now have two gardens to tend, so be careful what you wish for!). I had to trust that our finances would be enough to cover the increased expenditure. They have. I have had to trust in myself in completing the second year of my studies, which I have.

I am so lucky to have such a wonderful tribe of women walking beside me, who believe in me and support me. A loving family who tolerate my quirks (!) and who support me in my ventures. My second book was released to the world this summer - I had to trust it would be well received, and it was.

So I sit here in the local park on a warm autumn day, surrounded by fallen leaves. Today is my eldest boy's 22nd birthday. This last week, he was in hospital after an abscess erupted in his cheek, and he needed surgery. I had to trust he would be fine, and he is. My youngest is looking at universities for next September. Am I ready to let him go? I am also trying to embrace the changes of perimenopause and what this chapter ahead will mean, both for me and for women as a whole. I am reading, exploring, talking to others and sharing experiences.

My nest will soon be empty, I know. How will that shape me, I wonder? I need to trust now more than ever. In myself. This midlife chapter will be challenging. I hope what I learn will help others face the challenge in a more empowered way.

With much love, as always,
Anna x x

<u>"You're turning into Grandma!"</u>

This is a phrase I often hear from my boys, usually accompanied by an eye roll and laughter, and usually when I have said or done something that my Mum says or does - pointing out beautiful plants, talking to birds in the garden or telling them an "interesting fact" which they don't find at all interesting! My Mum often says that she sounds just like her mother when she has said something Grandma would say. I like to think of it as passing the ancestral torch, the continuation of habits and rituals rooted in generations of knowledge and wisdom (with some silliness thrown in), keeping family sayings and traditions alive. I will always look for "white horses" on the sea, the white foamy crests of waves offshore, as my Grandma did. In the age of Google, I still use her sponge cake recipe, and will ask my Mum why my bolognese isn't like hers rather than looking on the net. I wish I'd paid more attention when my grandparents told me family stories, and taught me about gardening and other such things, as I am now a grandmother and wish to pass the knowledge on.

This is why human females are the only species (other than Orcas) to have a post-reproductive lifespan. Through menopause and beyond, we support the next generation of mothers in supporting their offspring. Orca matriarchs will mind pods of infant whales while their mothers join the hunt for food. They remember the good spots for food, and teach the next generation where they are - sharing knowledge, guiding and teaching. As mothers, aunts and grandmothers, we older women can pass down our knowledge to the next generation, supporting our children/nieces/nephews in navigating their life journeys. Society sees the older woman as "past her prime", but we are far from it.

<u>Tuning into my inner Crone</u>

Crone is used in such a derogatory way in modern times. Even the dictionary says:

> Noun: Ugly old woman

(Think of the witch in Robin Hood: Prince of Thieves, a "typical" crone).

Simply put, a Crone is a woman post-menopause. In ancient times, the Crone was revered. She held the wisdom of the tribe or community, she was seen as the moral leader and possessed knowledge and skills for healing. Her presence was highly valued and celebrated (croneconfidence.com). As society evolved and the patriarchy took hold, older women no longer had a purpose. No longer able to bear children, and no longer allowed a voice, their wisdom and knowledge stayed silenced.

In 2022, this generation of women (aged 55 and over) made up 16.7% of the UK population (populationpyramid.net). Over 11 million Crones! Women who have lived their lives, raised families, have careers and relationships, studied, read, created, loved and lost, faced hardships and overcome challenges. Think of all that collective knowledge and wisdom! I think also of how they were kept small, made to experience and endure so much in silence, feeling alone, feeling trapped maybe. Going through their life stages not knowing what was to come or how to manage it. I feel so lucky that I have a community around me where curiosity and questioning is encouraged. We can access so many other Crones to ask about their experiences and seek guidance, exchange ideas and what has worked for us. I am also lucky that I have been introduced to my Inner Crone (or inner wise woman, or older self). In a coaching session with the wonderful Lisa Pascoe, pre-pandemic, she encouraged me to visualise her; her surroundings, her clothes, her features. I can see her so vividly. Long silver hair left wild, she wears a purple dress and silver jewellery. Her hands have spots of paint on them, or sometimes soil from the garden. She is surrounded by colour - paintings, fabrics, plants, candles and crystals. She has calming music playing, or it is quiet to allow the sounds of nature to be heard. She lives in a wooded area, overlooking a body of water. There is a porch with large, comfortable chairs overlooking the water.

By sitting and tuning into her, I can access the wisdom of the life she has lived. She is my inner knowing.

This may sound a bit "woo-woo" to some of you, but I guess it's similar to a gut instinct. When you know something deep down but don't want, or aren't ready, to hear it. We all have inner wisdom passed down through generations of wise women. Our grandmothers may not have been teaching a tribe or being revered by the village, but they passed their knowledge to their children and ultimately, some of that trickled its way to us.

Another wise woman who I revered growing up was a teacher I had in junior school. She was the last teacher I had before moving on to secondary school. Mrs Harvey. Oh, I loved her! She was vibrant and fun and creative, wore bright clothes and flamboyant accessories. She had silver-blonde, frizzy hair, and she was fabulous. She was the teacher who cast me as Joseph in our production of Joseph and his Technicolour Dreamcoat, and I got to wear her multi coloured blazer for my costume. During junior school, I was bullied by other girls, but having her as my teacher gave me some pleasure during these years. I wish I had known her as an adult, to learn more from her.

She was not your typical teacher or older woman. She was beautifully herself and wasn't afraid to stand out. What I love is seeing older women now expressing themselves creatively, dressing boldly, doing things that they want to do which spark their fire. And I love seeing them share their passions with the world to inspire others. Creating communities, passing on their knowledge and skills, their wisdom. We may not be doing it around a campfire anymore, but we are still here.

The modern Crones are taking back their power.

It's about time.

<u>4th November 2022</u>

Chatting with my cousin this week, we talked about our not-so-little ones flying the nest. Her eldest daughter, 23 at time of writing, now lives in London and is teaching. Her youngest daughter is 15 and has said she wants to study history at Durham University. She spoke of her excitement on their behalf, and of what this next chapter could hold for her - travels, adventures, and it got me thinking. After being a Mum for 22 years, surely now is the time for me to be as excited, to be making plans. What am I afraid of, in letting my boys go? Is my fear for them, or for me?

My eldest left home at the start of the pandemic, and returned home when his relationship broke down. He is in a new relationship now, and I don't feel as anxious for him as I do for my youngest who will be heading to university next autumn. I don't know where my anxiety is rooted. There are financial worries, naturally. There are worries about his safety; will he make friends easily? He's not as "street smart" as my eldest, will he be taken advantage of? Will he hate it, but feel he has to stick it out? Distance from home. Not seeing him each day. Not feeling like I'm part of his life anymore.
Ok, my fear is for me, isn't it.
I have been building a life for myself, slowly, doing things I enjoy, but still with my boys and my husband at its core. And it is important to have a life for you which does not depend on another person. I have been like a chameleon in the past, taking on the likes and interests of others without really considering my own needs and wishes. Now will really be the time to build on these wishes and dreams, time to bring them to fruition in some way.
Why does this feel scary?

<u>2nd January 2023</u>

2023, how are you here already? Some thoughts on the arrival of a new year:
I don't subscribe to the "New Year, New You" BS. There is nothing wrong with the existing you! You are enough, exactly as you are. The world needs more of your light, so continue shining bright, exactly as you are, quirks and flaws and all.

Be gentle with yourself, there is no need to rush into January with resolutions and new projects and commitments. We are still in winter, energy is low and beating yourself up for lacking motivation will start a downward spiral of "I'm not good enough."
Take your time.
Sow the seeds of what you hope to achieve in the year ahead, but don't jump in until it feels right for you. There is no rush to accomplish anything.

<u>5th March 2023</u>

I am realising that it is all going to coincide - transition to menopause, where my hormones will be even more out of whack; empty(ish) nest, my children stretching their wings and exploring the world without me; realisation that my parents are older and that one day I will be without them; realisation that I may have less life ahead of me that I have already lived.

How do you get your head around and come to terms with all of this?
Where do you even start?

Hormones. I have been trying to learn as much as I can about perimenopause, so I can be prepared and try to understand why I may feel certain things. Sophie has been an invaluable contact. As a menopause coach, who has experienced the process, you couldn't wish for a better woman to have in your corner. She has taught me so much, and I was shocked at how little I knew! We don't just have oestrogen and progesterone to worry about, oh no.
Oxytocin - the love hormone, which floods our systems to reinforce bonding with our newborn child and gives you that beautiful sated feeling after sex, dips in perimenopause. It can lead to us feeling detached in relationships, a sense of isolation, that no one gives a toss about whether we are here or not.
I have felt this very strongly over the last year or so, in fits and starts. I have felt lonely in my own home, that my family wouldn't even notice if I took myself off (at least not until the laundry piled up!). I have not attended social events and thought "it's ok, they won't even realise I'm not there." I have talked myself into dark places, convinced myself that I wouldn't be missed. That maybe things would be better without me.
I'm not needed as I once was - my children aren't excited that I'm home, they don't shout "Mummy!" and run to cuddle me. My marriage has also shifted, from being very physical to us seemingly just living in the same space. Our work patterns don't facilitate much time together, and we tend to socialise in different circles. What's going to happen when it's just us?

My mind can easily spiral, and I guess hormones aren't helping me when I feel disconnected from those I love. I know my menfolk love me. Only this weekend, my eldest, 22, came home from the pub at around ten thirty. I was in bed, but he came in and hugged me, and told me he loved me. Admittedly, he moaned when I refused to get up and make him boiled egg and soldiers, but we spent the next hour or so lying on my bed, chatting and watching daft videos online, laughing and giggling. My youngest, 17, tells me about his college work and what he's worried about. He often volunteers a hug.

I will very much miss having them around when they both fly the nest, but I will always be their Mum. My fears are irrational, and when I sit and write, I can unpick them as being so.

Another unexpected symptom I recently encountered - but had heard tell of - is that of rage. Unexplained, untriggered, but deep-seated rage. I had arrived at work, and everyone was asking me if I was ok.

"Absolutely fine."

But I wasn't, and I knew something wasn't right but I didn't know what. I felt angry for no reason. I was tense, snappy. After a couple of hours the feeling subsided. What the hell was that about?

According to the literature, oestrogen helps with the regulation of serotonin, the "feel good" chemical in the brain. With oestrogen levels falling, we have the symptoms of mood swings, emotional dysregulation, as well as sleep disturbance, low energy and lowered motivation (tick all of the above!). I have been taking antidepressants for many years - initially for postnatal depression, but found I struggled without them. These drugs work by boosting levels of serotonin in the brain. I guess this was pretty stable until my hormone levels started to dip. Mood swings I was ready for, but rage? Again, this is apparently due to fluctuating hormone levels. At peak oestrogen times of the cycle, if our cortisol level (the stress hormone) also peaks, and our serotonin level drops, this creates the perfect storm. Great.

When the feeling of rage had abated, and I was back in the office, I apologised to my colleagues and explained what I thought it was. At least I am not going mad, but it really did feel like I was losing control, and I didn't know when it would end or when it would happen again.

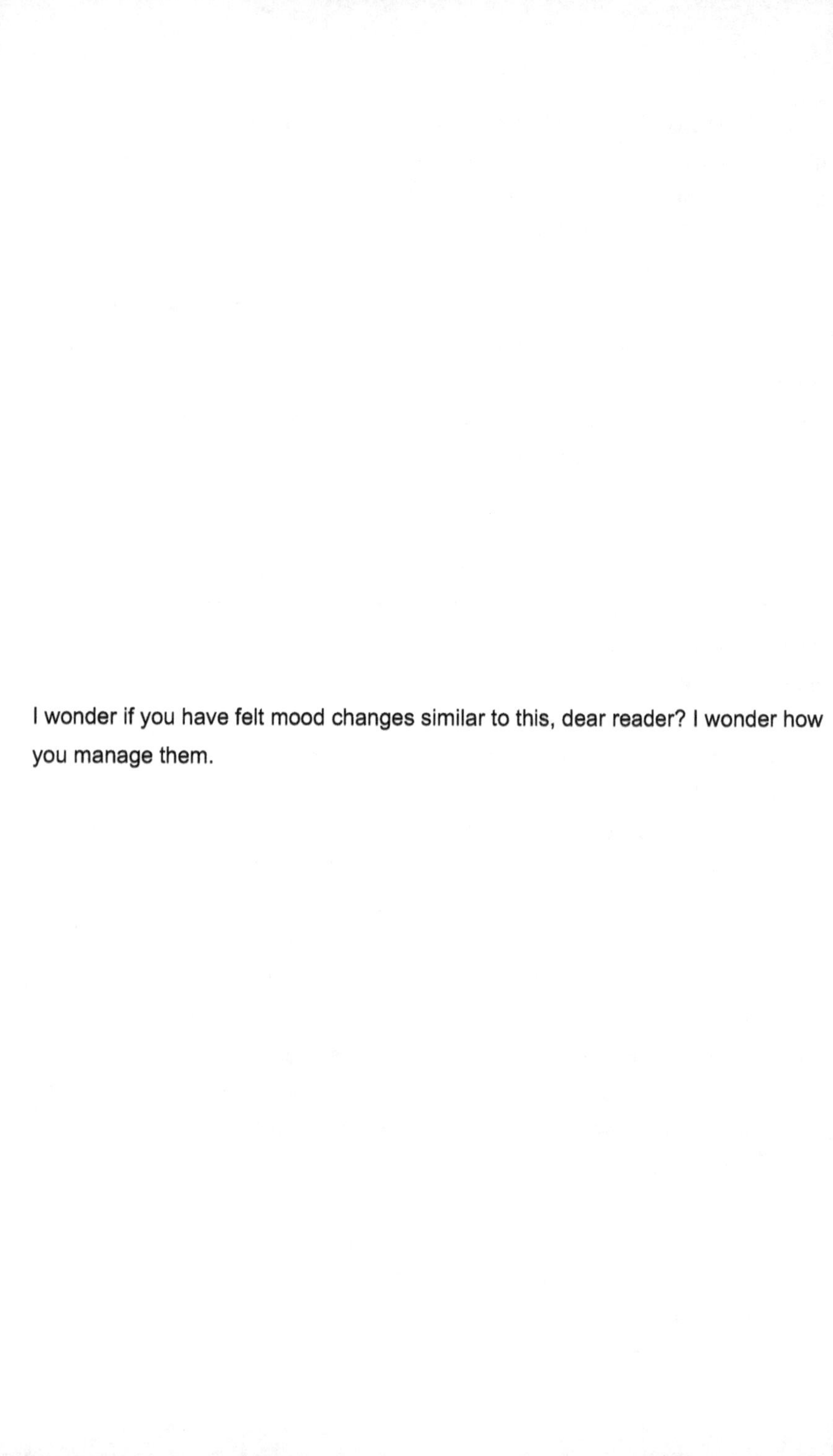

I wonder if you have felt mood changes similar to this, dear reader? I wonder how you manage them.

<u>18th April 2023</u>

I think it's the uncertainty that's scaring me the most. The "not knowing." What will life be like "after"?

After being a Mum.

When my youngest heads off to Uni in September, when it's just me and my husband. What if, after all these years of raising our family, we find there's no common ground? What if we have different lives envisaged?

I know that when I look ahead, I want to travel more. I want to start living, whether that's going to the theatre or seeing live music or seeing more of this country and beyond… I don't know what he has envisaged as a life going forward. I'm not yet fifty, and I know the next chapter will have challenges. I want a partnership, but still my own space. I want physical intimacy, I want to share experiences of sunrises and sunsets. I want lazy days reading by the sea. I want walks in the forest. I want to feel loved and adored, and maybe even worshipped a little. I want to feel that heat of passion again. I need it, to feel like… I don't know… the sacred feminine force in the relationship. I want to feel seen. And heard. I want to share my hopes and dreams without them being dashed.

I'm anxious about how menopause may change me, the emotions that may surface. The Rage inside me. How will it manifest itself? Will it be destructive? Am I going to shatter my bubble into a million pieces? By just wanting to be heard?

<u>19th April 2023</u>

I don't understand where the anger swells from. The Rage.

After a night where I struggled to get to sleep, and experienced a vivid dream about my husband having an affair, infecting me with HIV and me being forgiving and understanding (what does that even mean??) I woke up with a chest feeling tight and a pressure in my head like it was about to implode. I could barely speak to my family for fear of just shrieking at them. I took myself for a walk before I had to log on to the computer for work. I wanted to shout and cry, and I have no idea why. After an hour or so, the pressure subsided, but agitation remained. According to my period app, I am ovulating.

How can this shift be so much, mentally and emotionally? It felt like I was losing my mind and my world was about to shatter.

Apparently, these feelings are not unusual (thank you Sophie for the reassurance). So why does no one tell us? And if you have experienced a trauma in your life, such as a sexual assault, or have been living in "fight or flight" mode, the change in hormone levels will uncover a shitload of anxiety, fear, anger and more that we may have repressed or suppressed for decades. Maybe this explains why my initial gut emotional responses are those of a seventeen-year-old Anna rather than those of a wise 48-year-old woman? I have made the decision to seek counselling before more big changes occur. Before my son leaves. Before my job changes. A space to work through what comes up ahead of the storm hitting.

<u>19th May 2023</u>

I am home after a lovely few days on the Isle of Wight with my folks. It has become an annual getaway - me, my parents and my brother. Although we don't really live that far away, 30 minutes on the motorway, this feels like the only quality time I get to spend with them. It can feel tricky at times, as we are now four adults rather than "parents" and "children" as such, and we hold differing views on the wider world. Having said that, we are very close and it is a safe space.
I was worried about The Rage coming to the surface (thankfully it didn't!) and we had a great time exploring. If you know the Isle of Wight, then you'll know how beautiful it is. Shanklin Chine is stunning with its waterfalls and giant ferns growing through the gorge. Long sandy beaches with crystal clear water. Tennyson Down with its amazing views. The botanical gardens. We walked A LOT, my Mum and brother indulged in their love of photography, with stunning results. The house we stayed in was in a quiet area, with a beautiful garden oasis - it was stepped up into a hillside, a real evening suntrap. I got to share real conversations with my brother over (a bit too much) whisky and "old skool" tunes, an evening I will treasure.

It was also an emotionally hard week. I boarded the catamaran on the Saturday morning to travel across The Solent, and I cried. Tears of relief (not work for a week), exhaustion (after a manic few weeks at work), and worry about what drama may ensue in my absence at home. Meeting my family on the other side, my Dad got out of the car to open the boot. "You ok?" he asked. I shook my head as he gave me a hug. "You are now."
On the Tuesday evening, it all hit me. This is the problem with stepping away from reality. You relax. Your mind isn't distracted by the normal daily grind. Your brain has space for other things to creep in and you can't avoid them. Cooking myself some supper that evening, the tears came and they wouldn't stop. I was done.
But I wasn't alone.

I will admit, I was anxious about coming home. What was I coming home to?
Laundry, as it turned out.
Nothing had changed in my absence, and now it feels like I haven't been away. Back to cleaning, the food shop tomorrow, work on Monday, The old routine. Having had

this time away from it, I know it has to change going forward. I need to feel more nourishment from the day-to-day, otherwise time will pass by and what will there be to show for it?

<u>25th May 2023</u>

It's an unmooring.

Uncertainty.

Not knowing what is real, almost.

Wondering how things will pan out, ruminating on the worst case scenario.

Questioning every thought and feeling.

All-consuming.

Exhausting.

Not knowing who I will be when I wake in the morning - the Rageful Bitch, the teary mess. Will I feel like I'm drowning? Or will I have a day where I actually feel like me?

What does "me" even feel like anymore?

Am I feeling angry or sad, or just numb?

Disconnected.

Acting a part in my own life, being what others expect, while behind the mask I am crumbling away leaving only the empty shell.

Navigating Menopause: an alternative to Google articles (blog post)

I wanted to write something about menopause and women reaching midlife, and how even now we are supposed to "stay in our box". I read other posts about navigating menopause, and it started making me angry (surprise! Perimenopause!). They were all quite fluffy, about this being a "transformative stage" and "a new chapter", as well as how to foster "more satisfying and supportive partnerships", but what appeared to be lacking was the drive to fight against the status quo when it comes to society's expectations and moving toward what they truly want.
So, here are my thoughts from my experience so far…

Perimenopause has turned my brain upside down and inside out. Less of a transformation, more of an unravelling. Everything that had seemed stable and constant is now seemingly shifting under my feet, and I don't know where to hold for security. I am questioning everything, from my career to my parenting (which now is as a Mum to two grown-arsed men, both adults but with their own issues) to my marriage.
I have put 25 years into my career, and I do love my job and my colleagues, and am now coming to the completion of my Masters. However, looking ahead I am wondering whether this is what I want to do for another 20 years. Do I want to continue working all that time? As the main breadwinner for the household, I have felt until now that I don't have a choice, but that has made me resentful. There are other things I want to do with my time. I want to travel. I want to rest. I'm so tired of being depended on and having to do what is right for everyone else.
I am very aware that changes in my hormones may be fuelling some of what I'm feeling - there's the feeling detached from people we love as oxytocin levels decrease. There's the feeling low and tearful, as well as the physical symptoms - hot flushes, headaches, lack of energy. On the other hand, all the articles I have looked at talk about lack of libido… If only! Mine appears to have gone the other way, and that is also fuelling my current feelings. How can you foster intimacy when you haven't had sex or any kind of physical relationship for years? Being involuntarily celibate is one of the most difficult things I am having to navigate, and this feeds the

cycle of feeling unwanted and detached, fuels feelings of not being good enough, and feeds into my body image issues (which have been life-long).

All the articles talk about communication with your partner, about talking things through and "navigating menopause together". What happens when they're seemingly not interested? Or when they become defensive whenever you try to share how you feel? It makes you not want to talk in the first place.

Approaching menopause feels like approaching a fork in the road. If I keep on the current path, I know the journey ahead, but I don't know if I want to continue along that route. If I veer off, I will be driving blind, with no map or compass, and no idea where I'll end up or how I'll get there.

I see lots of posts about midlife being this liberating, empowering time where women can find their true voice and their true path. And for me that is partly true. It has certainly caused me to think about what I want going forward, but I still feel stuck. And it is easy to stay in the rut, because that's what we're conditioned to do - be the good girl, the good wife and mother. Put everyone else before yourself, make sure everyone else is happy. Don't make too many demands as you'll be seen as difficult. And we certainly can't say we want sex, only sluts demand sex. We shouldn't express a hunger for anything, as that is "unfeminine", whether it be for success, equality, attention, affection, recognition. So how are we supposed to express our true desires?

One thing perimenopause is showing me is that I am not as healed as I thought I was, and I have a lot of shit still to work through. Writing my books was just the start of peeling back the layers, it seems, and there is still a way to go. So, if you want to read some articles about how navigating menopause is as easy as talking openly with your partner, expressing your feelings and having them support you with exercise and positive words, Google can help you there. If you want to share a raw and less fluffy journey, watch this space, and please do get in touch if anything resonates with you. I am sure it's not just me.

<u>5th June 2023</u>

Well the weekend wasn't exactly as planned…

I had booked myself a long weekend off work as Hubby was going away with his friends. I had booked to go to a gig with a friend, there was a work's retirement meal, I'd planned to see friends, booked a photoshoot.

Then Hubby gave me Covid.

Annoyingly, he felt well enough (and was past five days of symptoms) to go away on his trip. I cancelled my plans. I was furious! I've avoided Covid for three years (quite a feat, working in a hospital!), and then it comes along on the one weekend where I had made plans for me.

Another thing I had wanted from the weekend was some time, some headspace. Be careful what you wish for, I had that in spades.

In between the dizziness and the naps, I had no distractions from my whirring brain. By Sunday morning (yesterday) I had to get out of the house, so at 8:30a.m., I drove to a quiet beach to just sit. There were already a few young families about, an older couple having a swim, groups of friends with paddleboards.

I felt so lonely.

I was overwhelmed with the feeling of not knowing who I was anymore, I didn't know where I belonged. Didn't know which of the roles I played was the real me, if any of them. I drove a couple of miles to where my grandparents' ashes are buried, and while folks were inside the church for Sunday Service, I sat on the grass next to their headstone and sobbed.

"I don't know what to do."

<u>11th June 2023</u>

This weekend, my brain has been kinder to me. Less frazzled, less berating, less angry.

I spent an entire Saturday sitting in the garden reading, and my Sunday started strong with an al fresco breakfast and a wonderful massage.

While eating my breakfast, I listened to a podcast from The King's Forum about discovering and developing your superpower. It talked about harnessing the pain from previous trauma, and really going deep to unlock patterns you may be repeating in your life. This in turn helps with finding who you really are under all the layers of survival and how we think we should present ourselves to the world. What we settle for when we could be living to our full potential.

I realised I have barely scratched the surface.

In my first book, I reflected on how my relationships went from one to the next, to the next. I never gave myself the space in my twenties and thirties to find who I was without the trappings of a relationship. I never left room to explore how to make myself happy, I always depended on them to do it for me. I always thought that they held the key somehow. I began new relationships in a place of vulnerability and wanting to be loved, and I didn't really explore how I needed that love to look. And when the initial honeymoon phase wore thin, I didn't know how to maintain myself.

In my second marriage, I had a second child within two years of being together. I threw myself into my roles as mother, wife, step-mum, and took on new challenges at work. I met a new friend when I was feeling overwhelmed. This offered me an escape from the daily grind, exciting opportunities. The chance to be someone else. It became a distraction from a reality I didn't know how to address. My friend had ideas about how I should address things, but I wasn't ready. I didn't know myself yet, who I truly was. I could see I was beginning to change, more confident at work for example, but more isolated from a wider circle of friendships. I had become blinkered, sucked into their version of my life.

When I cut myself off from that particular friendship, which had become all-consuming, I met other women who were supportive and empowering, with no other agenda than that. I began to see myself differently, I realised I had something to share with others and that's when I began writing. I know I am a different person to who I was before the pandemic. I wax lyrical about rewilding, connecting with myself and the life I truly want. Except, I am not yet living a fully authentic existence. It still feels aspirational. Over recent months, I have looked outside again for validation that I am enough - as a Mum, as a friend, as a nurse. In particular, as a woman. I have lost my inner spark. Last week, two good friends indulged a whim of mine to have a woodland photoshoot, the theme being Reclaiming Crone. I have already written about crones being the wise women, and with perimenopause in full swing, I wanted to do something to mark my intention of taking back my power as an older woman. The setting was gorgeous - ancient woodland and ferns, the sun setting giving a beautiful golden light (we won't mention the midgie bites!). As she started shooting me, Debbie looked at an image on her camera and said "you are just so fucking beautiful!" And I knew she meant it. I nearly cried, because I hadn't heard it for so long. I realise now that I have been relying on others to validate my beauty, wanting to be told rather than just knowing it within myself.

And that's the pattern.

I have to stop relying on others to validate me, and getting upset when it doesn't come. I have to stop seeking reassurance from others that I am enough. I have to believe it. Know it. Use it as a daily affirmation.

Just because my children are grown and spend less time with me, it doesn't mean I am not good enough as a Mum.

Just because my husband doesn't want physical intimacy, it doesn't mean I am not a beautiful, sexy, desirable woman.

Just because I don't know all the answers at work, it doesn't mean that I am not a bloody good nurse.

Just because I'm not a social butterfly, it doesn't mean I am not a good friend.

And just because my brain is like a rollercoaster with hormones and my emotions are all over the place, it doesn't mean I am not capable.

I have a lot of shit to process. It's going to be hard. I can't avoid myself anymore because I can't waste the second half of my life by not being me. I need to figure out who I am when all the roles are stripped away. I need to think about what I want from this one, wild, beautiful life. I need to know whether this mirrors what I have and what needs to change.

And it's terrifying.

<u>27th June 2023</u>

Hemmed in.
Suffocated.
Caged, like a bird desperate to spread its wings only the bars are restricting any movement beyond what her keeper will allow.
Maybe it's the recent oppressive heat we've had on the south coast of the UK, maybe it's a shift in my hormones, or maybe this is how I actually feel?
Who fucking knows anymore!

I'm really hoping counselling will bring some clarity, some distinction to what is real and what is not. How do I even know which thoughts are actually mine and which come from my Peri friend, my inner good girl (wanting to keep everyone happy) and my inner critic (wanting to scupper me whenever she can under the guise of keeping me safe)?
How do I tease them apart? I suppose I'm lucky that I have a degree of insight to know that not all my thoughts are true, that feelings are transient, and I'm not going to have the same thoughts and feelings at different times of the month. That's helpful. Equally, it doesn't help when trying to navigate and pin down what I actually want and need.
I have a tattoo on my arm depicting a bird flying free from its cage. I want to be that bird, but I don't know how to fly free - or where to fly to. All I know is that today I feel suffocated by where I am at. I want to breathe, without stealing everyone else's oxygen. And that's the crux of the matter. I'm so worried about hurting other people, people I love, that I won't stretch my wings further than my cage.
At least, not today.

Can we talk about sex (in menopause)? (Blog post)

What happens to our sex drive during menopause? Again, a frustrating search through various articles via Google leaves me annoyed. Apparently, we should expect our libido to drop at this time of life, and various sources tell us that this is how it is.

We well know that menopause is a natural phase in a woman's life, signalling the end of reproductive years. Alongside the hormonal changes, menopause can also bring about shifts in sexual desires and experiences. I want to learn more about the impact of menopause on sexuality, common challenges faced by women, and how to address this in the bedroom.

Because not all of us lose our sex drive. Some of us - me! - are wanting sex, at times more so than ever before, and it's a difficult one to navigate.

We know that our hormone levels change - oestrogen and progesterone decline, leading to physiological changes which may reduce our sex drive. With lower oestrogen comes vaginal dryness which can cause pain and discomfort. We experience fatigue, mood swings, hot flushes, and these can impact too.

In my search, I did find one article, written in 2015 by Suzi Godson - she posed the question "is it normal to have high libido later in life?". She talks about how preconceived ideas and "pessimism" about menopause have a huge impact on women's libido during menopause - if we're told our sex drive drops off, is it a self-fulfilling prophecy? She also talks about how she was in a new relationship, and I guess that honeymoon period helps with sexual appetite. A study she cites, where 600 women chronicled their experiences between the age of 40 to 65, showed that women who stated sex was moderately or extremely important to them maintained an active sex life.

For me, sex has always been an important part of my relationships, in cementing the intimacy between myself and my partner, and this may be playing a part in my continued sexual desire. I have stated in a previous blog that I have become involuntarily celibate due to my partner's health and other issues, and it has been difficult for me to adjust to as we were always very active. Other kinds of intimacy have also dropped, not just intercourse. How do I/we claw it back?

Many sources talk about communication being the answer, and again this can be tricky in some partnerships. If your partner isn't open to conversations about the issue, what do you do? Sometimes, upgrading your vibrator isn't enough! Articles talk about "experimenting with other methods of intimacy", which is all well and good if you're both up for it. If you're the only one missing the intimacy, where do you or can you start?

I don't have any answers, these are just my musings on the subject. I am only 47. I enjoy sex (even if I'm not supposed to say so, as older women are supposed to stay quiet on this subject…). I miss sex, hugely. I want sex.
Is it just me?

Link to Suzi Godson's article:
https://www.irishexaminer.com/lifestyle/arid-20314898.html

<u>18th July 2023</u>

Today is a good day.

The last week or so have felt like a rollercoaster, and I never know how I'm going to wake up. Some nights I have hoped that I don't wake up. I have had some joyous moments - meeting our new granddaughter, for example, was beautiful. I spent time with friends, had a wonderful weekend spa break! I did notice it took me a while to actually relax (by the end of my first Pimms, oddly…). My brain wouldn't quieten, and I felt restless on the sunlounger by the pool. My body needed to adjust to not needing to be "on." We chilled, read our books, enjoyed the hottub. We ate good food (room service in bed, thank you very much!), and a thank you to the previous guest who hadn't logged out of their Netflix account! Anyway, having that space allowed my body and brain to recover, and I hadn't realised how much I had needed it. I have just kept going for too long, thinking I was giving myself space, but not really achieving it.

My final assignment for my Masters has been submitted, which will free up a lot of brain space. I have started seeing a coach to try and get some clarity ahead of big changes in my life. Even after all these years, and trying to move away from it, I am a real people pleaser. Through past (and current) relationships, making my partner happy; through motherhood, putting my children's needs first; at work, wanting to prove I'm capable and a "good" team member; through wanting to make my parents proud. I need to learn again how to set those boundaries and be true to me.
I just need to figure out what I want…

Spookily, a few people I know who are spiritual/energy healers have recently said the same thing to me:
"You don't don't need counselling, you need healing."
One of them said they could see my aura, that my energy needs to be brought back to myself. Another had seen me during her meditations and sent me a message asking if I needed any help (that didn't freak me out at all!). Now, dear reader, I do have a spiritual sense of being unsettled and stuck, and some of you may see this as being "a little bit too woo," but maybe they're right? They obviously sense something. Maybe it would add to the clarity?

As I said, today is a good day. I could have become entangled in someone else's drama this morning, but I chose to stick to my day off as planned. Shopping and a pub lunch with my younger boy. I bought a fire pit for the garden (I've wanted one for years). I am spending some time writing, listening to the bees on the lavender (I wish this book could deliver audio and aroma, as it's heavenly).

My hormones are calm today, no anxiety spikes or crying spells as I have had recently at work, so I am making the most of it. I am grateful for it.

<u>2nd August 2023</u>

Well, it's been a funny couple of weeks, dear reader (which feels par for the course this year!). The last few days I have felt much lighter - a well-needed weekend camping in the New Forest with a friend gave me some distance from everything that's been causing me anxiety, such as work and dynamics at home. We walked in the trees, chatted for hours about all sorts of things (including how mankind is on a path to self-destruction, how religion has possibly caused more harm to the world than good, to inventing a new drinking game involving Revels chocolates and whisky!), and generally just relaxed in each other's company.

I've returned home with a more positive mindset about things. I feel more secure in myself when thinking about my son going to university. I feel more relaxed about work, not thinking I have to prove or justify myself every minute. I feel more assured to make plans to live my life to meet my needs.

Another thing that has helped is starting coaching. At my last session, we focused on "people-pleasing". I grew up wanting to be a Good Girl, wanting to do the right thing and make others happy and proud of me in the process. In my first book, I talk about my Green Pig money box and how being told off for painting it the wrong colour triggered my need to conform. In coaching we explored other aspects of people-pleasing - changing my plans to accommodate others, not speaking up so as not to upset others. As a mother, I had to prioritise the needs of my children, but now? At nearly fifty, I can please myself, can't I?

Well, you'd think!

I still want to keep others happy, but am starting to make changes and make myself happy too, like having my weekends away with friends. The Good Girl behaviour is definitely still present, but I think I need to have a word with her, tell her that she can relax now and think about herself instead, think about what she needs to be happy. Or, as my coach said, I need a "Don't Give a Shit" button and I need to press it. Life is short. I want to live mine, for me, and be happy. Pleasing everyone else is not going to allow me to achieve that.

<u>7th August 2023</u>

What a difference 48 hours can make!
Friday was my last day at work before two weeks off. I was done. Exhausted. Brain fog, barely able to string a thought or sentence together. I went to yoga, which I struggled with. My body was not happy, but I managed to relax a little. Saturday included a much-needed three-hour nap. Sunday (yesterday) was amazing. I took myself to London on the train, and as I left Waterloo Station to walk to meet my friends, I felt so light! I had no pressure to be anywhere (we'd left the meeting time flexible as a group of us from all over the country were attending and Meg, who organised the meet-up, would be there all day). I could walk where I wanted, stop when I chose to. I was completely anonymous in the big city and no one paid me any attention.
Meeting with my friends was just so lovely - some of them I had only met before via Zoom, so to be able to sit around a table and chat about anything and everything was just... amazing! We talked about life challenges, creative identity and ventures, pets, cults, bee-keeping (life goal!) and we all just got each other. No judgement, just acceptance for who we are, what we do, where we are now. I felt whole.
I have had many conversations recently about where I'm at in terms of my worries for the future, empty nest, do I still want what I've got. I actually have an amazing life. I am surrounded by people who I am so grateful for. They see me, accept me, love me. There's been a shift in my mind about my life going forward. It's mine for the living, and not everyone will approve or keep up, but it's my life. Days like yesterday make me so fulfilled. More like this please!
I just hope this mind-shift lasts...

<u>29th August 2023</u>

Ok, let's talk about the impact of broken sleep…

After having a wonderful two-weeks off work, I was feeling pretty good. I'd had a long weekend in the West Country with a friend full of exploring, good food and lots of laughs. I'd spent time with friends and family, had an amazing crystal reflexology session, and a much-needed massage to round the fortnight off perfectly. We also adopted a rescue cat, Lily. I was feeling so positive!

Back to work with a bump, a busy five days, and an unexpected change in sleep pattern. Struggling to get to sleep, waking in the early hours, and then oversleeping. I could easily say "hormones", but is that really all it is? On two mornings, Hubby got up for work (before 5a.m.) waking me over the weekend, my older boy was out for two nights and I can never settle until he's home. The cat was a dickhead on two of the early mornings - I swear she'd dropped some acid or something, racing around and meowing at 3a.m., shaking her maracas like it's carnival time!

I also started helping the younger boy get his bits together for university, the first of the dreaded (by my bank account) trips to Ikea. The time for him to leave is fast approaching. So maybe it's not just hormones - although night sweats are a bitch. Maybe my subconscious is mulling over the new reality on the horizon. Maybe I've been busy distracting myself from what's coming. The next chapter. Maybe I'm not as ready as I thought I was.

Or maybe it's Mercury in retrograde and I can blame the universe!

What I do know is interrupted sleep exacerbates so many other issues that come with perimenopause. Tiredness makes brain fog much worse (just ask my colleagues). It increases irritability and lethargy and reduces motivation. In my case, this week I have noticed my anxiety has been worse and little paranoid thoughts have crept in. I have been more sensitive to the moods of others, thinking if they're pissed off it must be because of me. It has made me less sure of myself at work, and made me feel less connected with loved ones. Even the cat.

I'm hoping this is temporary, another phase on the rollercoaster. Let's hope so.

<u>12th September 2023</u>

Dear 18-year-old Anna - you'll never guess what?! I went clubbing on Saturday night!! (Your reaction is probably the same as our 18-year-old son's, full of incredulity and embarrassment at the thought. Or maybe not?).

The reason for the excursion into night-time Portsmouth was a celebration of us completing our Masters this summer (you will have just received your A-level results… We never did like physics, did we?). I went for a lovely meal with a few good colleagues who had supported me through the three years, but when I thought about how to celebrate, I really wanted to go dancing. I haven't been dancing for so long! I haven't set foot in a nightclub for about 16 years, and I wanted to experience that freedom. Now, the nightclub scene has changed quite a lot, so choices were limited (we're no longer kicked out at 2a.m.) but we plumped for PopWorld where they play a good mix of music - cheesy wedding style, as well as the classics. In the end, just myself and one other went to the club. My dear friend, just retired, early sixties, loveably bonkers. We almost fell at the first hurdle as we didn't have ID on us (seriously?!) but they took pity on the oldies and we got in.

I really didn't know what I was expecting. I know in the last year or so, you have fallen out of love with mainstream clubs (hardly surprising after you were assaulted). Is that why I stuck to a corner to dance in, so no one could come up behind me? Maybe. It was a relatively small venue with a good mix of people, and we were definitely the oldest ones there. That was fine. Everyone loved my friend! Dancing with her, smiling, chatting to her - and why wouldn't they? She just let herself go and danced, not caring who was watching or what they thought. She looked totally free. As for me, I couldn't quite get there. I was very conscious of others around me, watching other groups so relaxed and playing with the music. I was very aware if men looked my way, but equally felt invisible as an older woman. Not confident enough to completely let go. Or not feeling safe enough to do so? It takes a long time for us to feel safe in crowded spaces again, and maybe my subconscious was being vigilant to keep me safe.

That feeling of being invisible is a strange one, and is not new to me. I have written before how, when women reach a certain age, they fall off the radar in society. Past our usefulness, we should now blend into the background.

Listen to me, my darling. I have spent far too long keeping quiet and doing the nest for everyone. I am now nearly fifty and am only just starting to reconnect with myself - with you. Promise me you will shout, make your wants and needs heard. Don't become invisible. Follow your path, put yourself first. If you don't, seeds of resentment will take hold and your voice will become choked. You will reach a point where you feel angry, and just want to scream, "THIS IS WHAT I WANT, WHY WON'T YOU LISTEN TO ME?!" And then you'll be a mad, bitter woman who is being demanding and selfish and inconsiderate in the eyes of others.
Darling girl, I want you to have a life fully lived. Be fulfilled. Be so, so happy. Don't stay small to keep others happy. Be brave. You are an incredible young woman with the world before you. Take it by storm.
I love you x x

<u>23rd September 2023</u>

No one tells you how hard this part is. You know the day is going to arrive, but nothing prepares you for it. Darling Anna, if I think back to where we were five years ago, you longed for the time when you would have space. When our teenage boys were driving us mad, when relationships were so strained it hurt.
"It won't be forever."
We wished it would be over, that time would fast forward to them being older. And now they are.
Tomorrow starts a new chapter, with our youngest heading off to university. As I write, he's upstairs (supposedly) packing his clothes and other bits from his room. In the living room in front of me are two Ikea bags and a storage box full of bedding, towels and kitchen bits ready to load in the car. In twenty four hours, I will be leaving him on the campus to drive home without him.
Do mothers ever feel ready for this moment? Surely I'm not alone in feeling such a mix of emotions? Can people just wave their kids off happily, without feeling that void? When our older boy moved out of home at the start of the first pandemic lockdown, emotions were different but it still hurt. And I missed him desperately. Then he came home when his relationship broke down, and I had a useful role to play (I thought) in being there to help put the pieces back together.
It's hard to go from being the centre of their world to having to watch from the sidelines. To not know the details of their day. To no longer be the first one they turn to. Taking that step back and letting them go. Our youngest has been more of a home-bird, not spending every minute with us but just being there. I won't be saying goodnight to him tomorrow when I go to bed. He won't be here when I get home from work on Monday. Or Tuesday. Or any day.
Chatting with a friend last night, he said, "you have given your whole life. It's time to take what you want. It's Anna's time. It's exciting. The world's your oyster." And I know he's right. We have spent two decades ensuring everyone else is catered for, happy and cared for, and now we have the time and space to turn that to us.
Curating the next chapter will be exciting. It's also fucking scary!
I'm no longer "Mum" first and foremost.
I'm Anna.

And I need to find out how she needs to be nurtured and nourished. What will feed her soul and bring her fulfilment. Because, Anna of five or six years ago, you more than deserve it.

<u>19th October 2023</u>

We're midway through October and it finally feels like autumn. Leaves are turning, the weather is certainly more seasonal and my need to prepare for hibernation is very present.

This week, I have been off work with a pesky cold. Work is so busy at the moment, that little voice has had a field day laying on the guilt. I haven't had the mental energy to fight the Inner Critic, and paranoia is creeping in - they think you're faking, they think you're lazy.

I've been resenting myself for having no energy, and the resentment seeps into other stupid thoughts. Resenting the cat for only giving affection to my husband, not wanting to curl up on my lap while I lay under my blanket. Resenting my husband for being so attentive to the cat - MY cat - when he hasn't shown me much physical affection for years. Resenting the fact that even now, we are struggling financially and had to ask my parents to help my son with money for university. Feeling like a failure no matter how hard I try, it's never enough.

Feeling isolated even in my family home. Feeling I can't share how I feel because no one will understand, or care. Feeling a lack of physical contact, that disconnect from loved ones. I can't remember the last time I had a hug, but it feels like a very long time ago.

I am trying to rest, physically. And I am trying to remember that these thoughts will pass. They are temporary, like the seasons. No storm lasts forever - it has to break. And there will be sunshine to follow, I'm sure.

<u>2nd November 2023</u>

On October 28th, the world lost a Friend. The actor Matthew Perry died in his home in America, thought to have drowned in his hot tub (although the post mortem was inconclusive). Matthew, who I have never met, has been part of my life for nearly thirty years. He played the character Chandler Bing in the sitcom Friends, and was instantly my favourite character. We slowly learned about his addiction struggles over the years, and watched his physical appearance change with each season as his repeated battles played out. My youngest son also fell in love with the show growing up, and we spent a wonderful day at FriendsFest (a festival, you guessed it, about Friends) a few years ago looking at sets and taking silly photos. We even have regular "Friends Trivial Pursuit" contests. The show has been a constant throughout my adult life. For me, it provided a comfort blanket when I was down, familiarity in times of uncertainty, a soundtrack in the background of daily life. Something I could watch without having to work hard to focus, chewing gum for the brain. But it was so much more.

My son messaged me when the news broke in the UK, around 1:30a.m. on the 29th. He thought it was a hoax to begin with. We spent the afternoon of the 29th together in his university digs watching Friends, him showing me posts and reels on social media. We shared in our sadness that Matthew Perry was gone.

I think I was taken aback by how sad I felt. It was genuine grief over a man I felt I knew well but didn't know at all. I read his memoir earlier this year - a heartbreaking read about his life and struggles, about how he never felt he was enough. He himself said in his book that he would like to be remembered for the help and support he gave to others who also struggled with addiction, but that he would probably be remembered for Friends. He set up rehab foundations and gave back so much. No one will ever know the truth about why his life was cut short at 54. He was alone, I believe.

I spent a couple of days feeling very sad and numb. Maybe it was grief for Matthew. I allowed myself to be with the feelings rather than distract myself. Maybe the sadness and grief was for more. Mourning other losses that I hadn't allowed myself to sit with - the move into a new phase of motherhood and what I leave behind, working to accept a new phase of marriage (will I grow to accept it? I don't know), the loss of my role as a lover. Taking the next step in my career, accepting a different role that doesn't yet fit comfortably. Accepting that I am moving into a new phase of life as a woman and what I no longer am.

Sitting with sadness is not easy! I have always managed to avoid or distract. It's uncomfortable, but maybe a little discomfort is needed to encourage me to shift position.

I am sad that Matthew Perry is no longer with us, but I am so grateful he has been in my life.

<u>15th January 2024</u>

It's a New Year! Halfway through the first chapter already. I have managed to avoid the "New Year, New You" onslaught as I don't believe midwinter is the time to bw putting extra pressure on yourself to "be better" - especially as we are pretty damn fabulous as we are.

Something I have noticed creeping in recently is a nagging inner voice. I know who the voice belongs to, someone I broke ties with pre-pandemic. A friendship that had become toxic over the years, impacting on other relationships in my life and causing me excessive anxiety. I would continuously second-guess and question myself, and for several months after I broke ties, I struggled to trust myself, trust my judgement. I had ignored my own inner voice for so long, I couldn't hear it. And when I did hear it, I couldn't trust it.

Lately, their voice has been creeping back in, especially when I feel I have not accomplished something to the best of my ability (self-judgement, anyone?). There are little things that used to make me anxious, such as what I wear. During our friendship, they introduced me to vintage styling, and I loved the dresses, the headscarves, the accessories. But they made such a point of making me feel "less than" one day, when I decided to wear a more relaxed style, I felt I had to up my game to meet their approval.

Lately, I've become more concerned about what I wear. This weekend I am going to London with my lovely friend to see Cabaret at The Kitkat Club (we are very excited!). I asked her today what she was going to wear.

"Ummm, clothes!" she replied, with a laugh.

Why am I so worried about what to wear? For my friend's approval? So other theatre goers approve? To prove something to my ex-friend?

I think it's odd that earlier in 2023, when I was at my most confused and mentally upside-down with my hormones, their voice didn't use that opportunity to return. It waited until things were more settled and I was starting to feel more secure in myself.

So I ask myself - what am I trying to sabotage?

The inner voice I hear is me, my thoughts, maybe echoing what my ex-friend has previously said, but it is my thought I hear. I need to acknowledge that voice, but equally, I don't need to listen to it or give it extended airtime. I can counter it with facts, with evidence that I am good enough. That I can wear what the hell I want! This is the year where I embody who I really am. Not a "new" me, but the real me.

<u>30th January 2024</u>

<u>HRT and Me…the journey so far.</u>
If you have followed my story, dear reader, you will know that 2023 was quite the year in terms of emotions and getting to know myself. It was certainly an education! Something I had to learn "on the job." I thought I'd try to summarise what I have learned about my hormones, HRT and perimenopause in case you are curious or are struggling too.
I thought that I had a fairly good understanding of my cycle and menstruation. I remember when I was in junior school finding a book in my local library called "Have You Started Yet?" which was all about periods. I pored over this book, fascinated and also excited about starting, feeling that I would then be a "grown up." My period started when I was 12, I think. We were on a family holiday and had just sat down in the restaurant for dinner when I felt it. Of course, I was wearing a white dress, but thankfully nothing leaked through.
I was over the moon! That didn't last long…
My periods through secondary school were awful. I fainted a couple of times at school. My Mum had to collect me numerous times from the nurse's office. Or I'd have to take days off to stay in bed with a hot water bottle. As soon as I was sixteen, I took myself to the G.P. to get the contraceptive pill, to hopefully ease some of the discomfort. I stayed on the pill until I was 24, and quickly fell pregnant with my eldest son. Back on the pill between pregnancies, my youngest arriving four and a half years later. I can't recall whether I took the pill again, but later opted for the Mirena coil (an intrauterine device impregnated with progesterone), and for seven blissful years, NO PERIODS!
In my early forties, I decided that I should give my body a break and go hormone-free (in terms of contraception). I had lost touch with my cycle and was aware that I was approaching the age of menopause. Initially my periods were regular, they weren't as heavy or painful as in my early days. Then at some point, things changed. They began arriving earlier than expected, lasting longer. By the end of 2022, my cycle was 21 days with a six day bleed. It was exhausting.
Now, what I hadn't been aware of was the interplay between these hormones and other neurotransmitters (chemicals in the brain responsible for mood, cognition and

pleasure, to name but a few roles), or that oestrogen wasn't only produced by the ovaries.

Why aren't we taught this?

Oestrogen plays an important role in how we regulate our body temperature, in immune response, metabolism, reducing inflammation throughout the body, keeping joints and muscles healthy. So when we begin perimenopause and our oestrogen levels fluctuate dramatically, we get hot flushes, joint pain and stiffness, and weight gain.

What was a real "ta-dah!" moment for me was discovering that oestrogen (which is produced in the brain as well) also affects the neurotransmitters serotonin, dopamine and noradrenaline. Serotonin is the chemical associated with mood and anxiety, and antidepressant medication works by boosting levels of serotonin in the brain. I have been taking an antidepressant for years, but noticed that there were days when my mood would be lower, I would be more anxious, I wouldn't have the motivation. And then it would pass. Depression doesn't come and go, so I knew it wasn't my Old Friend returning. Apparently, when levels of oestrogen drop, this in turn can cause a drop in serotonin levels. Serotonin also plays a role in sleep, pain and appetite, as well as mood and anxiety.

Lower levels of oestrogen will also lead to lower levels of dopamine. This is the pleasure chemical (and what social media thrives on, getting that next hit), a reward system in the brain triggering a hit of pleasure and heightened arousal. Lower dopamine levels will impact negatively on our memory, concentration level, how we focus, as well as our motivation.

Brain fog, anyone?

There are days when I can barely string a coherent sentence together! Joining this mix is lowered levels of noradrenaline, which is a chemical responsible for alertness, focus or attention, as well as enhancing memory formation and retrieval. Is it any wonder I felt like I was losing my mind? And that's just oestrogen!

Progesterone tends to decline first in perimenopause, and doesn't have the peak and trough fluctuations we see in oestrogen. It just drops and that's that. In terms of the monthly cycle, it's progesterone which prevents our womb lining from building up, but it also helps with sleep as it's a natural sedative. It can help with mood too, so lower levels can often cause depression, mood swings, anxiety and panic. It also impacts another neurotransmitter called GABA. GABA is like a soothing balm for our brain. It's an inhibitor and regulates over-activity which will in turn help with feeling irritable and anxious, and can help with concentration and sleep. It may also impact on our self-control, impulsivity and disinhibition, as well as sensitivity to over-stimulation.

When I think back to this time last year, I can recognise just how much I was impacted by these symptoms. I was irritable and highly anxious, I was seeking validation. My sleep was atrocious, I was exhausted. I booked some sessions with a menopause coach (the wanderful Sophie) and suddenly everything fell into place. I saw my G.P. (I'm lucky that my local surgery has a female G.P. with a special interest in menopause) and we discussed my symptoms and my options. I was still a little reluctant to go full in with HRT, so opted to have progesterone replacement initially. As there was a waiting list for the Mirena coil, I had a progesterone depot injection instead - a three monthly injection of the hormone. The difference this made was incredible.

I was no longer going mad! It was like a fluffy blanket had settled around my brain. That was in late spring/early summer, and things did improve mentally. I was still getting brain fog, occasional hot flushes, and my sleep fluctuated.

In November, I went back to my G.P. and I started oestrogen replacement on December 1st. I use the Oestrogel topical gel, two pumps each morning rubbed into the skin. Again, I felt the benefits quite quickly. I feel more balanced mentally, less irritable, less anxious, able to concentrate a bit better. And less like I want to tear my skin off because I feel so horny! Thank goodness *that* settled!

Unfortunately, I had to wait several months to get my Mirena coil (my surgery stopped providing the service, so I had to go through our local sexual health clinic). I finally had it inserted on January 3rd. Not the most pleasant experience ever.

The downside I am dealing with now is that my period started on Christmas Day and I am still bleeding. Yep, nearly six weeks, folks (I've had the coil checked, all is well and no infection). I guess because I have higher levels of oestrogen now, the womb lining is building more. When I started having the progesterone injections, my periods went from six days every three weeks to a two-week bleed every eight weeks. I'm hoping as the coil settles that things will even out (and maybe I won't have a period for a while... please?). It's definitely swings and roundabouts, but mentally I am in a much better place with the HRT than I was earlier last year.

I feel lucky that I had an experienced coach to reach out to for support and a G.P. with a special interest, who took me seriously. As you saw in my introduction, not all of us are so fortunate in terms of support from the NHS, or know where to access the information. I will be including information about where to find support at the end of the book.

<u>6th May 2024</u>

Dear reader,

I have not forgotten you over recent weeks, I promise! My aim is to have this book out in the world by October 2024.

The last few months have been busy, but less rollercoaster-like. I have been getting my head around what I have written - re-reading the first draft today has made me realise just how far I've come and how much I was not myself this time last year. Physically, my peri symptoms are more manageable - and I haven't bled for about three weeks!!!!!! I still wake most nights at around 2:30a.m., and often struggle to wake in the mornings, but my joints ache much less. Mentally, the brain fog is worse when I'm tired. The anxiety feels less intense overall, the paranoia is pretty much gone, and I can recognise my down days as being temporary.

I am taking time for me. Earlier this year, I signed up for a twelve-month creativity coaching programme with the wonderful Meg Kissack, called Your Rebellious Year. I have been able to have protected time to explore what feeds my inner critic and some amusing ways in which I can shut her up! I have looked at ways to grow into my most creative self, and ways in which I can make time for things I find nourishing. I am less berating of my need for decompression time, when I need to watch familiar TV shows without having to focus, where I can scroll on my phone or play games, giving my brain time to regroup and settle. I do not need to be productive all the time. I can choose how I use *my* time for *me*.

I have spent time with friends, whether out for dinner or chilling on the sofa with a cuppa. Yoga and sea-dipping when I feel up for it, but not beating myself up if I don't. My son has nearly completed his first year at University (where has that time gone?), and part of my brain wonders "what was all the fuss about?"

Life continued.

Nothing imploded.

Some things haven't changed that still need to be addressed, but maybe the timing isn't right yet. The next hump in the rollercoaster could be just around the corner, but I keep telling myself "it will all work out, because it has to," one way or another.

This book is my journey so far. I know perimenopause isn't done with me, and tomorrow something may well derail me. But tomorrow isn't here yet. Sitting at my

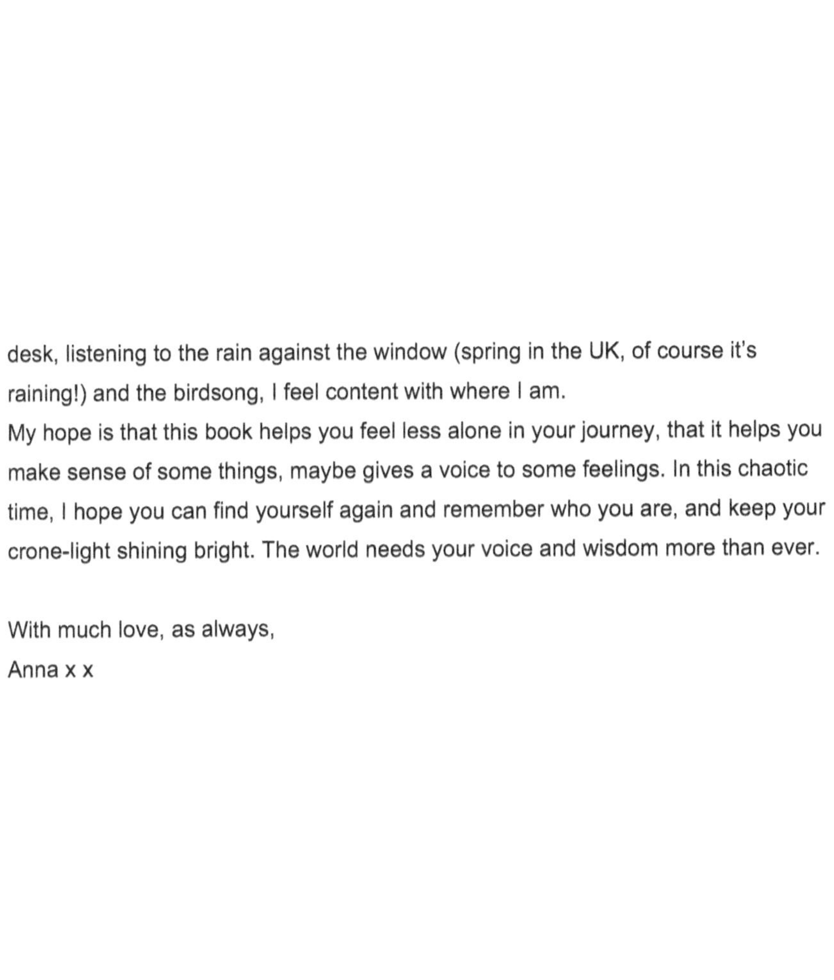

desk, listening to the rain against the window (spring in the UK, of course it's raining!) and the birdsong, I feel content with where I am.

My hope is that this book helps you feel less alone in your journey, that it helps you make sense of some things, maybe gives a voice to some feelings. In this chaotic time, I hope you can find yourself again and remember who you are, and keep your crone-light shining bright. The world needs your voice and wisdom more than ever.

With much love, as always,

Anna x x

Acknowledgements

Firstly, a huge thank you to you, dear reader, for buying my book! In those moments where the doubts crept in and I thought "no one will want to read this," you have kept me going.

Thank you to Sophie Cartledge (Hormones on the Blink) and Harrah Murray (The Beautiful Mind Coach) for your time and coaching, bringing me back from feeling I was going insane.

Thank you to Dr Louise Newson (@menopause_doctor) for continuously sharing your wisdom in a way which is accessible.

Thank you to the women who have supported me and cheered me on in my writing. To Hannah Roper for her encouragement and for running The Female Creative Brunches, where I have connected with other fabulous women. To Meg Kissack for being generally wonderful and for curating You Rebellious Year and The Rebel Social, a much needed space and again, a platform through which I have met so many inspirational women. To Anna Sansom, for inviting me to write in a different genre and trusting my work for her anthology.

To Debbie Fowler, for indulging me in photoshoots to reconnect with myself.

To Mel Barrett, for being my oldest friend and me sounding board (on the rare occasion our diaries match!).

To Chloe, Russell and Myanna, for keeping me sane at work.

And to Amy Shutler, my work-wife, yoga-buddy and all-round "couldn't do life without you" girl. Love you.

<u>Resources</u>

Sophie Cartledge, Hormones in the Blink
Menopause & hormone health training provider
Empowering a more positive menopause and hormone health experience through interactive, educational workshops and training.
@hormones.on.the.blink (Instagram)
www.hormonesontheblink.com

Dr Louise Newson
Menopause Specialist
@menopause_doctor (Instagram)
@balancemenopause (Balance app, in app stores)
www.newsonhealth.co.uk

Hannah Murray, Beautiful Mind Coaching
www.beautifulmindsupport.co.uk
@the_beautifulmindcoach (Instagram)

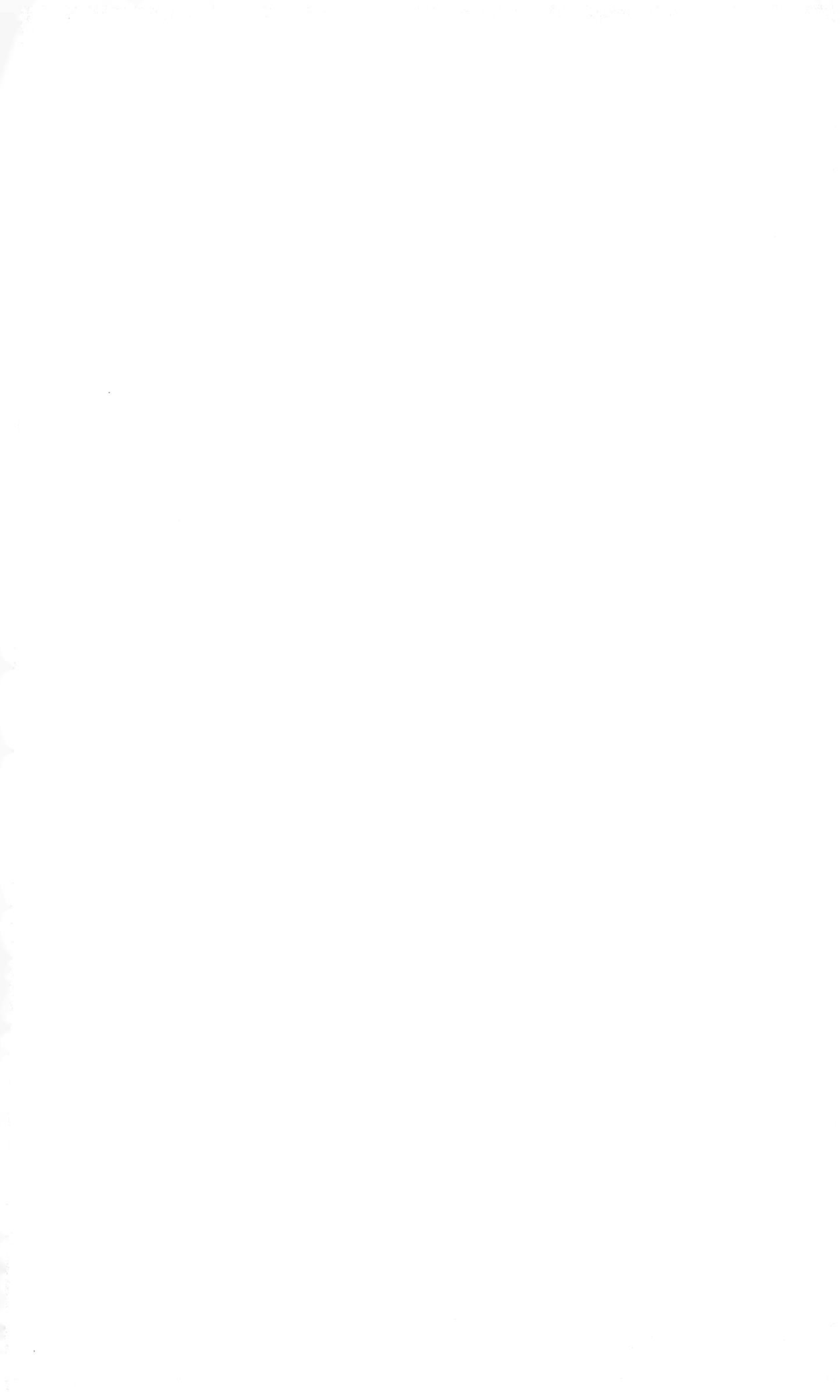

www.ingramcontent.com/pod-product-compliance
Lightning Source LLC
Chambersburg PA
CBHW031334250726
48656CB00005B/2116